# My Bulletproof Diet Recipes: Healthy Recipes to help you stick to the Bulletproof Diet

*by Jessy Smith*

**Disclaimer:**
The information provided in this book is designed to provide helpful information on the subjects discussed. The publisher and author are not responsible for any specific health or allergy needs that may require medical supervision and are not liable for any damages or negative consequences from any treatment, action, application or preparation, to any person reading or following the information in this book.

**Note: This Book is Not Written By Dave Asprey of bulletproof, but by Jessy Smith to help people looking for 100% Bulletproof Diet recipes to enable them stick to the diet plan.**

## Table of Contents

Herbal berries Serenade
Blueberry Light
Parsley Refresher
Deli' Mexican Meal
Zucchini grass-fed Beef Bake
Energy boaster coffee
Chocolate magic coffee

**Bulletproof Diet Approved Foods**

**Enjoy**

**Recommended Health & Fitness Bestselling Books**

## Introduction

The Bulletproof diet is seen as the healthiest way to eat as it's the only nutritional approach that works with the genetics of human beings to help them stay lean, energetic and strong.

Studies in biochemistry, Ophthalmology, biology, dermatology and other disciplines show that it's our modern diet, loaded with processed foods, sugar and trans fats, that is at the root of killer diseases such as diabetes, heart disease, cancer, infertility, depression, obesity, Alzheimer's, and Parkinson's disease.

This Diet is a healthful diet, an abrupt change and Elimination from the Standard American Diet (SAD). This is related to the Paleo/Caveman Diet with proof of Sustainable weight loss in a long term period. In this diet we have eliminated most of the Foods that enhance weight gain and bring to you healthy fat burning foods that would help you lose weight and stay healthy for a longer period. The Diet is designed to reduce body fat, enhance mental performance, and prevent disease while leaving you Satisfied and Energized.

The Bulletproof Diet is divided into:

## The Simple Bulletproof Diet

This Diet is specially designed to reduce your body fat, enhance mental performance and prevent disease while leaving you satisfied and Energized. In this Diet Plan you are advised to eat only when you are hungry and stop when you're satisfied, snacking is not an option here, so you are advised against it. Also, you are allowed to target 50% to 70% of calories from healthy fats which includes all the good fatty foods, 20% from Vegetables, 20% from protein and 5% from fruit or starch. For Optimum results you are advised to eat more of oil and Fat with Organic Veggies such as zucchini, lettuce, avocado, asparagus etc. And reduced fruit or starch intake to one to two servings per day in the evenings to avoid your triglycerides getting high.

## Bulletproof intermittent Fasting for Fat Loss and Focus

This Diet Plan makes it possible to lose fat easily while increasing mental Focus and energy without craving.

In this Plan, You start by consuming a cup of bulletproof coffee in the morning this would help increase your mental focus and increase your work energy for the day. Eat Only the Food listed in our recipes with high bulletproof rating to achieve optimum result.

## Bulletproof Protein Fasting

This Plan aids in the reduction of inflammation. You are advised to limit your protein intake to 15-25g for about two to three times a week. This would help cleanse and detox your inner-cells without any record of muscle loss. Also, you should consume a cup of bulletproof coffee to keep you full and energized throughout the day, take low carbs meals and high fats the rest of the day. To achieve optimum result, take the foods listed in our recipes with bulletproof rating from 2-3.

Here in this bulletproof cookbook, we have specially prepare some easy and quick mouthwatering recipes that would enable you follow through each and every one of this bulletproof diet plan easily. We've done our research and made sure that the ratio of foods we prepared fall into the bulletproof diet approved foods. So, be rest assured that all our recipes are 100% Bulletproof.

## The Simple Bulletproof Diet Recipes

Here we have prepared foods that are in line with this diet plan. This Mouthwatering, Quick and Easy Meal, will help you stick to the plan easily, you can substitute any of the recipes you don't like with related recipes shown in the foods to eat. Enjoy

## Delicious Meatballs

### Preparation time: 30 minutes approx.

### Yield: 4 servings

### What you need:

1 lb grass-fed red Meat
4 green onions, sliced thinly
4 teaspoons coconut oil
2 teaspoons sesame oil
4 teaspoons fish sauce
4 tablespoons coconut, shredded
Sea salt, to taste

### How to make it:

1. Combine all the listed ingredients in a large bowl excluding oils.
2. Make a mixture and roll the mixture with hand to make balls.
3. Heat oil in a skillet and cook meatballs in skillet until brown.
4. Now place foil in a baking tray and cook in oven at 375 degree F for about 25 minutes.
5. Serve and enjoy with your favorite Paleo friendly dipping.

## Vanilla Granola Cereals with Orange

**Preparation Time:** 5 minutes
**Cooking Time:** 30 minutes
Yield: 6 Servings

### What you need:

2 cups of Almonds (raw)

1 cup of pumpkin seeds (raw)

1 cup of sunflower seeds (raw)

1 cup of flaked coconuts

¼ cup of Chia seeds

1 tablespoon of vanilla bean (grounded)

1 ½ tablespoon of orange zest

½ cup of maple syrup (pure)

¼ cup of olive oil

¼ cup of apple butter

1 cup of apricots (dried, chopped)

### How you make it:

1. Preheat your oven at 275°F.
2. Pulse the almonds in your food processor until they have been chopped a bit.
3. Take a large bowl and add the almonds, pumpkin seeds, sunflower seeds, chia seeds, coconut flakes, orange zest, maple syrup, olive oil and apple butter.

4. Stir until the mixture is combined into a sticky, chunky batter. Take two baking trays and add some baking sheets to them. Pour the chunky mixture on to the sheets and flatten it a bit.
5. Bake them for 30 minutes in the oven or until it is golden brown.
6. Make sure to check after every 10 minutes and give it a stir to prevent it from sticking.
7. Take them out, add the apricots and let the granola cool off.

## Tasty Baby Spinach with Orange

**Preparation Time:** 10 minutes
**Cooking Time:** 10 minutes
Yield: 3 servings

**What you need:**

6 strips of pastured bacon fat

2 teaspoons of olive oil

4 pastured eggs (beaten)

½ cup of baby Spinach (lightly packed)

8 slices of apple

Salt and Pepper (to taste)

**How you make It:**

1. Take a medium-sized skilled and crisp up the bacon strips over medium heat in the olive oil.
2. Set them aside to rest on paper towels to drain their oil.
3. Once they cool down, chop them into bite-sized bits.
4. Take a small bowl and beat the eggs lightly.
5. Add the apple slices, torn baby spinach and salt and pepper.
6. Mix once more and set aside.
7. Heat up some butter in the skillet at medium heat.
8. Once the butter melts, pour in the omelet mix.
9. Watch them carefully and once the omelet starts cooking, fold it over. And let it cook some more.
10. Once it becomes golden brown, take it off the heat.

**Serve:**
Serve with some extra bacon bits and a small salad of bacon bits, apple and baby spinach.

## Tasty Bacon Bite

**Preparation Time:** 25 minutes
**Cooking Time:** 20 minutes
**Yield:** 4 Servings

**What you need:**

4 strips of pastured bacon fat

1 ½ cups of bell peppers (assorted colors, diced, peeled, deseeded)

4 pastured eggs

1/4 cup of baby Spinach (lightly packed)

1 tomato (small sized, diced)

1 white onion (diced)

Salt and Pepper (to taste)

**How you make it:**

1. Leave your oven to preheat at 350°F.
2. In a skillet or sauce pan, start cooking the bacon strips on medium heat.
3. Don't crisp them; leave them a little raw.
4. Add in the diced onions, tomatoes and peppers and sauté them in the pan with the bacon for 7 minutes or until they start to cook through then set aside.
5. Take a bowl and crack the eggs into it. Beat them lightly and season with salt and pepper.
6. Take a cup cake baking tray and line with silicone baking cups.
7. Spoon the bacon and vegetable mixture in each cup, half filling it up.
8. Take the bowl and pour the beaten eggs on top until the cup is almost full.
9. Bake them for 17 minutes in the oven or until the eggs look done according to your liking.
10.

**Serve:**
Pop out a bite sized omelet and enjoy warm. You can have more than one and pack the rest for lunch or breakfast some other day.

## Grass-fed Beef with Brussels sprouts

**Preparation Time: 25 Minutes**
**Yield: 4 Servings**

### What you need:

2 tablespoons coconut oil
2 tablespoons chopped onion
1 teaspoon ginger and garlic, paste
½ cup grated sweet potato, peeled and grated
6 ounces of grass-fed beef
3 ounces of Brussels sprouts, shredded
4 pastured eggs, cooked as per liking (1 per serving)

### How you make it:

1. Heat the oil in skillet and sauté onions in it.
2. Then add potatoes and cook for few minutes.
3. Once potatoes are tender, add the ginger garlic paste.
4. Give it a stir and add Brussels sprouts.
5. Add water to pan and cook on low heat for about 30 minutes.
6. Top with fried egg and enjoy.

## Tasty Chicken Soup and vegetables

**Preparation Time:** 25 minutes
**Cooking Time:** 10 minutes
Yield: 4 Servings

### What you need:

4 cups of water
Meat from one Pastured chicken (whole, diced)
1 cloves of garlic (minced)
1 onion (yellow, diced)
4 tomatoes (diced, medium)
1 zucchini (small, peeled, diced)
2 carrots (diced)
1 bay leaf
Salt and pepper (according to taste)

### How you make It:

1. Take a large pot and on medium heat, combine the water, chicken, onion, bay leaf, pepper and garlic.
2. Allow the water to come to a boil. Turn the heat down.
3. Place a cover on top of the pot and let it simmer for 2 hours or until the chicken becomes tender.
4. Uncover the pot and remove the bay leaf.
5. Now add the remaining ingredients and allow the soup to come to a boil again before reducing the heat again.
6. Place a cover on top and let the soup simmer for 20 minutes more or until the vegetable are tender.

**Serve:**

Serve hot with some steamed vegetables on the side or have as is.

## Crunchy pastured Chicken Legs

**Preparation Time:** 10 minutes
**Cooking Time:** 1 hour
**Yield: 4 Servings**

### What you need:

4 pastured chicken legs (quarters and thighs)
½ cup of almond meal
1 teaspoon of curry powder
1 teaspoon of cayenne
1 teaspoon of mustard (dry)
4 tablespoons of olive oil
Salt and pepper (according to taste)

### How you Make it:

1. Leave your oven to preheat at 350°F.
2. Take a baking dish and line it with some baking paper and set aside.
3. Take a large bowl and add the almond meal, curry powder, cayenne, dry mustard and some salt and pepper. Mix them well and then set aside.
4. Clean the chicken thighs and quarters and rub each piece generously with olive oil.
5. Crumb each thigh by rolling it in the almond meal mix you made. Make sure they are all coated well and give each one a light shake to remove excess almond meal.
6. Place them on the baking paper and pop the dish in the oven.
7. Cook for an hour or until the coating gets crispy. Test the chicken by piercing them with a skewer.
8. If the juices run clear, take them out, otherwise, cook for 10 minutes more then check again.

**Serve:**
Serve hot with some steamed vegetables on the side.

## Baked Sockeye Salmon with Lemon and Dill

**Preparation Time:** 20 minutes
**Cooking Time:** 20 minutes
Yield: 2 servings

**What you need:**

2 Sockeye salmon fillets (6 ounce each)
2 zucchinis (sliced thinly, lengthwise, halved)
¼ of a red onion (sliced thinly)
1 teaspoon of dill (fresh, chopped)
2 slices of lemon
1 tablespoon of lemon juice
Olive oil (extra virgin)
Salt and pepper (according to taste)

**How you make It:**

1. Leave your oven to preheat at 350°F.
2. Take two pieces of large parchment paper and fold each in half to make a crease down the center.
3. Now open the papers and place them on to two baking trays.
4. On one side of the crease, place some zucchini and onion slices, sprinkle some dill and place one slice of lemon.
5. Drizzle some olive oil on top and season with salt and pepper.
6. Place one fillet of salmon on top of the vegetables.
7. Drizzle the lemon juice on top and season with some more salt and pepper.
8. Now fold the other half of the parchment over the salmon and start rolling the two sides together to seal them.
9. You should end up with a crescent-shaped, lumpy package.
10. Make the other package in a similar manner and seal it in the same way.
11. Next, pop both into the oven and let them cook for 15 to 20 minutes or until the salmon starts going opaque. Discard the parchment once the salmon is cooked.

**Serve:**
Serve warm with some steamed vegetables on the side.

## Raspberries Pancakes

**Preparation Time: 15 minutes**
**Yield: 2 Servings**

**What you need:**

2 cups of coconut flour
2 cups almond flour
Pinch of salt
2 organic eggs
2 teaspoons of walnut oil
1 cup raspberries
1teaspoons baking powder
Honey (optional)

**How you make It:**

1. Mix the coconut flour, almond flour, salt, baking powder in a bowl.
2. Take another bowl and mix reaming ingredients
3. Combine ingredients of both bowls to make a batter.
4. Pour the spoon full of the mixture into preheated greased pan to make the pancakes.
5. Once the top gets bubbly flip to cook other side.
6. Serve with drizzle of honey.

## Bulletproof Coffee Recipe

**Preparation Time: 4 Minutes**
**Yield: One Serving**

### What you need

1 cup of brewed dark coffee, any local brand
2 tablespoons of grass-fed organic butter
1 tablespoon of palm oil

### How you make it:

Make your coffee using French press.
Dump the brewed coffee in to mug filled with butter and plum oil.
Stir and serve hot.

## Jessie' Butter Coffee Recipe

**Preparation Time: 5 Minutes**
**Yield: one serving**

**What you need:**

3 shots espresso
1-1/2 cup hot water
1 tablespoon of Kerrygold grass-fed organic butter
1 teaspoon of organic coconut oil

**How you make it:**

Pour the boiling water into the coffee mug and brew espresso in it.
Add in the coconut oil and butter.
Pour the mixture into the blender and blend for 30 seconds
Pour into the mug and enjoy hot.

## Non-Salted Butter Coffee and Palm Oil

**Preparation Time: 2 Minutes**
**Yield: One Serving**

**What you need:**

1 tablespoon of MCT palm oil
2 tablespoons of non-salted grass fed butter
1 tablespoon of coffee
1 cup of water

**How you make it:**

First boil the water in a pot on high heat.
Blend the entire listed ingredient in a blender until frothy.
Serve in to cups and enjoy.
Brew the coffee in water.
Add in palm oil and butter.
Mix the liquid in blender for about 20 seconds until it is creamy and no oil sits on the surface.
Pour in to the serving cups and enjoy.

## Natural buttered coffee

**Preparation time: 5 minutes**
**Yield: 2-3 servings**

**What you need:**

4 large tablespoons of high quality herbal coffee
2 cup water, boiling
1 tablespoon of coconut oil
Few drop of stevia
Few drops of vanilla extract
1 tablespoon unsalted butter

**How you make It:**

Pour the boiling water in blender and brew coffee in it.
Once the coffee brewed, add the coconut oil, stevia, and butter.
Pulse for about 30 second until a smooth texture is obtained
Just before serving add the vanilla extract and serve hot.

## Bulletproof intermittent Fasting Recipes

Here, we have prepared some delicious Recipes that would help you lose fat easily while increasing mental Focus and energy without craving. You are allowed to substitute recipes that fall under the bulletproof diet Approved Food. Enjoy!

## California, Kale and Sweet Potatoes

**Preparation Time: 50 Minutes**
**Yield: 4 Servings**

**What you need:**

1 large cauliflower, cut and cubed
5 sweet potatoes, baked
1 cup kale, chopped
4 bell peppers, chopped
3 small onions, chopped
1 cup coconut oil
1 tablespoon ground cumin
1 teaspoon ground coriander
3 lemon juice, squeezed
Sea salt & pepper, to taste
4 ripe avocados sliced
3 tablespoons of water

**How you make it:**

1. Preheat the oven at 350 degree F.
2. Bake the potatoes in oven for about 30 minutes.
3. Take a large pot and heat oil in it
4. Add bell pepper, onions, salt and black pepper,
5. Next, add kale and cook until ingredients get tender.
6. Next add in cauliflower and water, let it cook with lid on for 20 minutes.
7. At the very end add the baked potatoes and squeeze lime juice on top.
8. Let it simmer and then serve

## Delicious Eggs with Pastured Pork

**Preparation Time:** 10 minutes
**Cooking Time:** 20 minutes
Yield: 1 serving

**What you need:**

2 tablespoons of avocado oil
¼ pound of pastured pork sausages (raw, bulk)
2 pastured eggs
Black pepper (freshly ground, according to taste)
¼ cup of water
1 tablespoon of guacamole

**How to make it:**

1. Take a stainless steel biscuit cutter and grease it well with the avocado oil.
2. Place it on a plate and stuff it with the pork sausage meat.
3. Gently press the meat down until it is packed well in the biscuit cutter.
4. Take the eggs and break them separately into two bowls. Beat each one and set aside.
5. Heat some oil in a saucepan or skillet over medium heat.
6. Once the oil starts simmering, slide the meat, with the biscuit cutter around it, from the plate and into the pan.
7. Let the meat cook for a minute or two or until its edges start shrinking away from the cutter, before sliding the biscuit cutter off.
8. Cook for 2 minutes more before flipping. Cook the other side for 2-3 minutes as well or until it is to your liking.
9. Clean the biscuit cutter and this time, grease two cutters. Keep the saucepan on medium heat and heat some more oil in it.
10. Add the two cutters to the pan. Take the bowls and pour one beaten egg into one cutter. Add seasoning if required.
11. Now pour the ¼ cup of water into the pan. Avoid getting any in the cutter and do not splash on the eggs.
12. Lower the heat, put a tight fitting lid on the pan and let the eggs cook for 3 minutes or until they are done to your liking.
13. Slide a spatula under the cutter and lift the eggs, with the cutter around them, out of the pan.
14. Leave them to rest on a paper towel and gently slide the cutters off.

## Kale Salad with Avocado

### Yield: 2 servings

### What you need:

½ cucumber, sliced
1 handful **almonds**
½ head of **kale**
1 **avocado**
1 handful radishes, sliced
Sea salt, to taste
½ lemon, squeezed for juice

### How you make it:

1. Sauté (toss) the kale and avocado, using your hands.
2. Then add the radishes, cucumbers, and almonds.
3. Finally toss the salad with lemon juice and sea salt.

## Pastured Chicken, Caribbean-Spiced

Yield: 4 Servings

### What you need:

1 1/2 tbsp. fresh lime juice
2 fluid ounces rum
1 tbsp. brown sugar
1/4 teaspoon cayenne pepper
1/4 teaspoon ground clove
1/2 teaspoon ground cinnamon
1/2 teaspoon ground ginger
1 teaspoon black pepper
1/2 teaspoon sea salt
1/2 teaspoon dried thyme leaves
1 (3 pound) pastured chicken
1 tbsp. vegetable oil

### How you make it:

1. Preheat oven to 325 ° F (165 ° C).
2. In a small bowl, combine the lime juice, rum, and brown sugar; set aside .
3. Mix together the cayenne pepper, clove, cinnamon, ginger, pepper, sea salt, and thyme leaves.
4. Brush the chicken with oil, then coat with the spice mixture.
5. Place in a roasting pan, and bake about 90 minutes, until the juices run clear or until a meat thermometer inserted in thickest part of the thigh reaches 180 ° F.
6. Baste the chicken with the sauce every 20 minutes while it's cooking. All ow chicken to rest for 10 minutes before carving.

## Bulletproof Fried Eggs

### Yield: 2 servings

### What you need:

4 pastured eggs
1 Tablespoon nut almond butter
½ Teaspoon sea salt
1/8 Teaspoon marjoram
1/8 Teaspoon pepper
½ Teaspoon parsley
2 Teaspoons red wine vinegar

### How you prepare it:

1. Break the pastured eggs into skillet over half Tablespoon melted almond butter.
2. Add spices and cook until whites are solid.
3. Place eggs onto serving plates.
4. Heat for two minutes, after melting remaining half Tablespoon of almond butter.
5. Stir in red wine vinegar and allow mixture to cook for another minute.
6. Pour over eggs.
7. Garnish with parsley and serve.

## Bullet Proof Beef Meatloaf

**Preparation Time:** 10 minutes
**Cooking Time:** 45 to 55 minutes
Yield: 4 servings

### What you need:

1 pounds of grass-fed beef

1 onions (red, medium, chopped)

2 pastured eggs

2 cloves of garlic (minced)

½ a red pepper (peeled, deseeded, chopped)

¼ cup of cilantro (fresh, chopped)

½ cup of parsley (fresh, chopped)

1 tablespoons of coconut oil

1 teaspoons of cumin (powder)

Salt and pepper (according to taste)

### How you make It:

Leave your oven to preheat at 350°F. Take a baking dish and line it with some baking paper and set aside.
Take a large bowl and add all the ingredients, including the eggs, onion, ground beef, the herbs and garlic and cumin powder. Season with salt and pepper and mix the mince together to combine well. Once everything is combined, take the baking tray you prepared earlier and place the mixture on it.

Pop it in the oven and cook for 45 minutes or until the meatloaf starts turning golden brown. Use a skewer to pierce and test the center of the meatloaf. If it isn't cooked, bake for 10 more minutes.

**Serve:**

Serve hot with a light salad or steamed vegetables. You can also freeze them for later use.

## Crunchy Coconut Pancakes

**Crunchy Coconut Pancakes**

**Preparation Time:** 5 minutes
**Cooking Time:** 10 minutes
Yield: 1 Serving

**How you make it:**

3 tablespoons of coconut flour
¼ teaspoon of baking powder
3 pastured eggs
1 scoop of Vanilla Protein powder (pea, rice, whey or any other preference)
¼ cup of Almond Milk.

**How you make it:**

1. Take a small bowl and add all the ingredients together.
2. Whisk until you have a smooth, lump free batter.
3. In a skillet or sauce pan, heat up some coconut oil on medium heat.
4. Take a ladle and spoon a helping of the batter you have prepared.
5. Use the back of the ladle to spread the mixture slightly.
6. Cook on one side for 2 minutes or until the pancake feels firm and golden brown then flip it on to the other side and cook for 2 minutes more.

**Serve:**
Let the pancake cool a bit then drizzle some honey on top or eat warm.

## Tasty Pastured Chicken with pineapple

**Preparation Time: 20 minutes**
**Yield: 5 Servings**

**What you need:**

3 pastured chicken breasts
4 rings of pineapple
1 tomato
2 tablespoons lime juice
Salt and pepper
4 tablespoons olive oil
4 tablespoons of water

**How you make It:**

1. Heat oil in skillet and cook until brown.
2. Sprinkle salt, pepper and water cook with the lid on for about 10 minutes.
3. Once the steam cooks chicken and make it soft.
4. Grill the pineapples on grill and then add to chicken.
5. Next, add lime juice, tomatoes and cook for 10-15 minutes at medium heat.
6. Once done serve and enjoy.

## Tasty Tacos

**Preparation Time: 15 minutes**
**Yield: 2 servings**

**What you need:**

4 paleo based tortillas
2 tablespoons salsa
2 pastured eggs
Salt and pepper

**How you make It:**

1. First, top tortilla with salsa.
2. Heat oil in skillet and cook eggs to make scramble.
3. Divide the scramble egg mixture between the tacos.
4. Serve and enjoy.

## Grass-Fed Beef Stew

**Yields: 6 servings**
**Preparation Time: 50 minutes**

### What you need:

12 ounces grass-fed beef, cubed
1 cup sweet potatoes, cube
1 can tomatoes, cubed
2 large onions
½ cup olive oil
2 red bell peppers
6 cups water
4 cloves garlic, minced
2 teaspoons red chili powder
4 teaspoons lemon juice
Salt and pepper, to taste
Paleo bread, side serving

### How you make it:

1. Heat oil in crock-pot and add beef, potatoes, tomatoes, onions, bell pepper water, garlic, chili powder, lemon, salt and pepper.
2. Cook on high heat for about 40 minutes until thick gravy formed
3. Serve with paleo bread if liked.

## Pastured Egg butter coffee

**Preparation Time: 5 Minutes**
**Yield: One Serving**

**What you need**

1 cup of organic coffee
3 pastured eggs yolks
1 teaspoon of Erythritol
Pinch of sea salt
3 cups of water

**How you make it:**

Through the coffee beans in French press along with 3 cup of water gave it a stir, cover it and let it sit for 5 minutes.
Once, the coffee is ready dumped it in a blender along with yolks.
Blend it for few seconds and then add remain ingredients
Let it blend for another 40 seconds and then pour in to the cups and enjoy
If your coffee seems too thin, add few more yolks.

## Pastured Egg yolk butter coffee

**Preparation Time: 5 Minutes**
**Yield: One Serving**

**What you need:**

1 cup coffee about 250 ml
360 ml water hot water
3 Pastured egg yolk (beaten)
1 teaspoon stevia
Pinch of cinnamon
Pinch of sea salt

**How you make it:**

If brew our coffee using French press or any other way you like.
Dump the eggs in blend and blend slightly
Next add in coffee, and the remaining ingredients
Give it final blend of 40 seconds and serve

## Chocolate Organic grass-fed butter

**Preparation Time: 5 Minutes**
**Yield: One Serving**

**What you need:**

1 teaspoon of stevia
2 teaspoon of organic grass-fed butter
1 teaspoon coconut oil
2 shots of espresso
2 tablespoons of dark chocolate unsweetened
2 cups of water boiling
Few drops of vanilla

**How you make it:**

First take a blender and combine butter and stevia, then add in espresso and blend by combining all the reaming listed in blender.
Once froth mixture is obtained serve.

## Ultimate Butter Coffee

**Preparation Time: 5 Minutes**
**Yield: One Serving**

### What you need:

1-2 tablespoons homemade ghee
½ tablespoons Grass fed gelatin
8 ounces organic coffee beans, freshly grated
1-2 cup boiling water

### How you make it:

First place being water in a blender and add in coffee and blend until it is brewed.
Next, add gelatin and ghee.
Blend until froth.
Serve hot.

## Sumptious Sesame Green Beans

**Serves 6**

**What you need:**

3/4 pound fresh green beans
1/2 cup water
1 Tablespoon Almond butter
1 Tablespoon soy sauce
2 teaspoons of sesame seeds, toasted

**How you prepare it:**

1. In a saucepan, bring beans and water to a boil; reduce heat to medium.
2. Cover and cook until the beans are crisp-tender, for about 10-15 minutes; drain.
3. Add soy sauce, almond butter, and sesame seeds; toss to coat.

## Bulletproof Protein Fasting Recipes

We have made sure you enjoy your meals while you lose weight and keep it off. That's why we have prepared some delectable recipes to help you through this plan which aids in the reduction of inflammation. As usual, you are allowed to substitute the recipes with the bulletproof approved foods. Enjoy!

## Grass-fed Beef with Stir Fried Vegetables

**Preparation Time:** 10 minutes
**Cooking Time:** 15 minutes
Yield: 3-4 Servings

**What you need:**

12 ounces of Sirloin steak (boneless, sliced thinly, trimmed fat)

2 tablespoons of olive oil

1 clove of garlic (pressed)

¼ cup of burgundy wine

1 onion (yellow, cut thinly)

1 red pepper (deseeded, cut into strips)

2 stalks of celery (chopped)

4 ounces of carrots (sliced thinly)

4 ounces of mushrooms (sliced thinly)

3 tablespoons of lemon juice

Salt and pepper (according to taste)

**How You Make it:**

1. Take a large skillet and on medium heat, add the garlic, half of the wine and a tablespoon of oil. Sauté the beef for 5 to 7 minutes or until the beef starts browning.
2. Scoop out the beef and set aside.
3. Heat some more olive oil and sauté the red pepper, celery, carrots and onion for 4 minutes or until the onion becomes tender.
4. Add the remaining wine, mushrooms and lemon juice to the skillet.
5. Stir-fry all the vegetables together for 3more minutes.

6. Add the meat and stir-fry for another minute more before taking it off the heat.

**Serve:**
Serve hot with a good helping of the stir-fried vegetables on the side.

## Delicious Avocados with cilantro

**Preparation Time: 35 Minutes**
**Yield: 4 servings**

**What you need:**

4 avocados, peeled and pitted
2 limes, juiced
2 jalapeno peppers, diced
2 clove garlic's, minced
2 small onions, minced
2 tomatoes, diced
1 tablespoon of fresh cilantro, chopped
Sea salt and ground black pepper to taste

**How you make it:**

1. Take a bowl, and add in avocados and squeeze lime juice on top.
2. Now, mash the avocados by fork.
3. Add in the jalapeno, garlic, onion, tomatoes, cilantro, salt, pepper and mix well. Serve and enjoy.

## Tasty Two Ingredients Pancakes

**Preparation Time: 20 Minutes**
**Yield: 2 Servings**

### What you need

4 large pastured eggs
3 bananas
1 teaspoon of baking soda

### How you make it:

1. Beat eggs with hand beater and add mashed bananas.
2. Beat slightly to make a paste and add baking powder.
3. Heat oil in pan and cook the pancake, serve and enjoy.

## Chestnuts with Guilt Free Paleo Coconut Macaroons

**Preparation Time:** 30 minutes
**Cooking Time:** 12 - 15 minutes
Yield: 20 small Macaroons

### What you need:

2 pastured eggs (whites only)
½ cup of raw honey
1 teaspoon of vanilla extract
Lemon zest of 1 lemon
1 ½ cup of grated coconut
2 tablespoons of coconut oil
Salt (according to taste)

### Coating of the Macaroons:

3 ½ ounces of dark chocolate
1 teaspoon of coconut oil
1 tablespoon of chestnuts (cleaned, chopped)

### How you Make It:

1. Leave your oven to preheat at 350°F.
2. Take a baking dish and line it with some baking paper and set aside.
3. In a large bowl, combine the honey, lemon zest, vanilla, salt and the egg whites.
4. Use a whisk and mix everything until it becomes foamy.
5. Add the coconut oil and the coconut flakes and whisk again.
6. Set aside and let it rest for 20 minutes.
7. Take a tablespoon and use it to tightly pack a ball of the mixture and place it on the baking sheet.
8. Make similar balls with the rest of the batter.
9. Pop the tray into the oven and let it bake for 10 to 12 minutes or until the macaroons start turning golden.
10. Transfer them onto a wire rack and let them cool.
11. Use a double broiler and melt the dark chocolate and mix it with the coconut oil in a bowl.
12. When the coconut macaroons have cooled, dip one end in the chocolate while the chocolate is still hot.

13. Sprinkle some chestnut on top and let the chocolate cool.

**Serve:**

Serve as is with some extra coconut cream on the side.

## Pastured Eggs, Spinach with Mushrooms

**Preparation time: 15 minutes**
**Yield: 4 servings**

**What you need:**

6 pastured eggs whites
1 cup mushrooms chopped
1 tablespoon coconut milk
1 cup baby spinach, chopped
Salt and pepper to taste
½ cup green onions, chopped
1 tablespoon olive oil for frying

**How you make it:**

1. Beat the eggs and combine mushrooms, coconut milk, spinach, salt, pepper, green onions in it.
2. Heat oil in a skillet and pour the mixture into the pan.
3. Let it cook for 5 minutes each side until eggs get firm.
4. Serve and enjoy.

## Butter Scallops

**Preparation Time:** 10 minutes
**Cooking Time:** 15 minutes
**Yield:** 3-4 Servings

### What you need:

2 tablespoons of coconut oil
½ cup of shallots (minced)
2 teaspoons of garlic paste (fresh)
2 teaspoons of ginger paste (fresh)
¼ cup of tomato paste
1 ½ teaspoon of garam masala
¼ teaspoon of cumin (ground)
¼ teaspoon of cinnamon (ground)
1 pound of sea scallops (fresh, cleaned)
8 ounces of coconut cream
Cilantro (fresh, garnish)
Cayenne pepper (according to taste)
Salt and pepper (according to taste)

### How you Make it:

1. Take a large wok and heat up the coconut oil on medium high heat.
2. Add the shallots and cook for 2 to 3 minutes or until the shallots start to soften.
3. Add tomato paste, ginger paste, garlic paste, garam masala, cumin, cayenne, cinnamon and season with salt and pepper.
4. Cook for 3 to 5 minutes, stirring constantly.
5. Add the scallops and the coconut cream to the pan and stir to combine everything and cook for 5 minutes or until the scallops are cooked through.

**Serve:**
Serve hot with some fresh cilantro sprinkled on top.

## Tasty Tomato Soup

**Preparation Time: 35minutes**
**Yield: 5 Servings**

**What you need**

2 tablespoons olive oil
2 teaspoons minced garlic
1 cup minced onion
1 cup tomato paste (you can make it at home my grinding the fresh tomatoes in blender)
2 liter pastured chicken stock
½ cup diced tomatoes
3 teaspoons dried basil
½ teaspoon dried marjoram
1 bay leaf
½ teaspoon dried oregano
1/3 teaspoon dried thyme
Salt and pepper

**How you make It:**

1. Heat oil in a skillet and sauté onions in it.
2. Once onions are translucent add garlic, tomatoes paste and cook for 5 minutes.
3. Add in the stock, marjoram, thyme, basil, oregano, bay leaf and diced tomatoes.
4. Bring the mixture to a boil and then cook for 30 minutes at low heat with lid on.
5. Once done serve and enjoy.

## Hemp Berry Smoothie

Yield: 2 Servings

**What you need**

1 cup frozen blueberries

3 tablespoons hemp seeds
2 tablespoons hemp protein powder
1 cup almond milk
2 pitted dates

1 cup spinach, kale or other greens

1 teaspoon cinnamon

1 teaspoon macademia

**How you make it:**

1. Blend all ingredients in a high speed blender.
2. Add more almond milk if the texture is too thick.

Enjoy!

## Herbal berries Serenade

**Yield: 2 Servings**
**What you need:**

1 cup water
1 cup raspberries (frozen)
1 apple (minus the stalk, chopped)
¼ cup cilantro/coriander
1 celery stalk
1 1/2 cup mild greens
1 cup of Ice

**How you make it:**

1. Place all the ingredients into blender and blend until mixture is a green juice-like consistency.
2. Add ice and blend again until creamy.

**Tips**

For the Mild green, go on, test this out with a small amount of strong greens too and feel the smooth, thick and delicious taste.

## Blueberry Light

Always refreshing and light. Good for sipping in the summer or while chilling in the beach.

### Ingredients:

1 cup water
1 cup blueberries (frozen)
1 apple (without the stalk, chopped)
¼ cup dill
1 celery stalk
1 1/2 cups mild greens
Ice

### How you make it:

1. Place all the ingredients into blender and blend until mixture is a green juice-like consistency.
2. Add ice and blend again until creamy.

## Parsley Refresher

Yield: 2 Servings

### What you need:

1 stalk celery
1 pear
½ cup fennel
1 cup parsley
1 cup greens of your choice
1-2 tbsp. lemon optional
1 cup water
Pinch sea salt
Add ½ cup ice

### How you make it:

1. Place all the ingredients into blender and blend until mixture is a green juice-like consistency.
2. Add ice and blend again until creamy.

## Deli' Mexican Meal

**Serves 2**

**What you need:**

1/4 cup chunky salsa
4 pastured eggs, poached
1/3 cup cheddar cheese, shredded
2 Tbs. sour cream
1/3 cup avocado, cut into chunks
2 Tbs. fresh cilantro, finely chopped
2 Tbs. olives, sliced

**How you prepare it:**

1. Cook eggs by poaching method.
2. Heat salsa in microwave or on stove, over medium high heat.
3. Place poached eggs on serving plate and top with salsa, sour cream, olives, avocado, parsley and cheese.
4. Serve

## Zucchini grass-fed Beef Bake

### Yield: 4 Servings

### What you need:

1 lb. ground grass-fed beef
4 zucchini, cut into 1/4 inch slices
1 cup chopped onion
Olive oil
1 cup chopped celery
1 cup sliced mushrooms
1 6oz tomato paste
1 t salt
2 cups shredded mozzarella cheese
1/2 t oregano
1/4 t pepper

### How you Make it:

1. Heat oven to 350.
2. Arrange zucchini in 13x9 baking dish.
3. Cook onion and celery in oil for 5 minutes, in a frying pan.
4. Add the ground beef, cook until it loses its pink color.

## Energy boaster coffee

**Preparation Time: 5 Minutes**
**Yield: One Serving**

**What you need:**

Few drops of stevia
2 cups brewed coffee, steaming
1 teaspoon of hazelnut, powdered
Pinch of sea salt
1 tablespoon of grass fed unsalted butter
1 tablespoon of palm oil

**How you make it:**

Pour steaming hot coffee in to blender and add in all the remaining listed ingredients
Blend for 30 seconds and then serve

## Chocolate magic coffee

**Preparation Time: 5 Minutes**
**Yield: One Serving**

**What you need:**

10 ounces hot black coffee, fresh grated
2-4 cups of boiling water
½ teaspoon chocolate extract (to taste)
½ teaspoon hazelnut extract (or to taste)

**How you make it:**

Pour fresh coffee into mug and pour boiling water on top. You can brew the coffee using hand held Frothier or French press.
Add in the extracts and butter, mix well.
Serve.

## Bulletproof Diet Approved Foods

### Nuts & Legumes

Coconut
Olives
Dates
Almonds
Cashews
Macadamia
Chestnut
Pine nuts
Brazil nuts
Dried Peas
Soy
Corn nuts
Soy Nuts

### Fruits

Pineapple
Tangerine
Grapefruit
Pomegranate
Apple
Apricot
Cherries
Kiwi
Figs
Nectarine
Orange
Peach
Pears
Plum
Lychee
**All Berries**
Cantaloupe
Raisins
Lemon
Lime

## Vegetables (Organic)

Artichokes
Green Beans
Carrots
Green onion
Zucchini
Radishes
Asparagus
Broccoli
Cauliflower
Avocado
Cucumber
Kale
Collards
Spinach
Cabbage
Lettuce
Fresh Corn
Elephant Peppers
Fresh Tomatoes
Onion

## Beverages

Green Tea
Butter Coffee
Fresh fruit juice
Pasteurized milk
Soy milk
Soda
Sports Drink
Nutribullet
Kombucha
Fresh coconut Water

## Oil & Fats

Grass-fed red meat
Coconut oil
Avocado oil
Cocoa butter and chocolate

Grass-fed butter, fish oil
Palm oil
Palm kernel
Raw almond
Raw macadamias
Virgin olive oil
Cashew butter
Grain-fed butter
Canola
Peanut
Margarine
Grass-fed bacon fat
**Dairy**
Butter (Grass-Fed)
Butter (Grain-Fed)
Skim milk
Cheese
Powdered Milk
Pasteurized non-organic yogurt
Pasteurized Non-Organic Milk
Evaporated milk

## Protein

Pastured Eggs
Grass-fed beef and lamb
Soy protein
Farmed seafood
Hemp protein
Farmed meat
Beans
Pasteurized dairy
Pastured chicken
Cheese
Trout
Salmon

## Starch

Cassava
Black rice
Potatoes

Wheat
Gluten-Free Powders
Buckwheat
Oats
Quinoa
Brown rice
Taro
Yam
Pumpkin
Carrot
Banana

## Spices and Seasoning

Apple Cider Vinegar
Sea Salt
Parsley
Cilantro
Cinnamon
Onion
Table Salts
Paprika
Nutmeg
Tofu
Mustard Seeds

## Sweeteners

Maple Syrup
Brown sugar
Cooked honey
Fruit juice concentrate
Coconut sugar
Glucose
Raw honey
Stevia
Erythritol
Agave
Sucralose (Splenda)

## Enjoy

If you Follow through the ultimate guideline provided in The Bulletproof Diet By Dave Asprey , And some of the Healthy and Delicious recipes we have prepared for you. You are going to be seeing great results in your body and health, because it is proven to work.

**If you enjoyed the recipes in this book, please take the time to share your thoughts and post a positive review with 5 star rating on Amazon, it would encourage me and make me serve you better. It'd be greatly appreciated!**

If you have any question or anything at all you want to know about this program, you can hit me up via mail thru jessysmith247@gmail.com I am always there to help you.

## Recommended Health & Fitness Bestselling Books

**The Bulletproof Diet: Lose up to a Pound a Day, Reclaim Energy and Focus, Upgrade Your Life** – NewYork Times Bestseller, Order it Here>> http://amzn.to/1Hs7Ec4

**It Starts With Food: Discover the Whole30 and Change Your Life in Unexpected Ways!** By Melissa & Dallas – NewYork Times Bestseller, Get it Here>> **http://amzn.to/1pwksD7**

Other Health Related Books You Would Like

## BOOKS BY BESTSELLING AUTHORS

**My 10 Day Green Smoothie Cleanse Protein Recipes: 51 Clean Meal Recipes to help you After the 10 Day Smoothie cleanse!**

The 10 Days Green Smoothie Cleanse is a Phenomenal Program created to help people lose weight in 10 Days. This program is so powerful and life changing, that lots of people have achieved weight loss.

However, it is sometimes difficult to maintain the weight loss after the 10 day green smoothie cleanse, and that's why we have prepared high-protein meals to Assist with weight loss after the cleanse. In this Book you'll discover lots of High protein recipes that are healthy, clean, and delicious!

**Get it HERE>>** http://www.amazon.com/Green-Smoothie-Cleanse-Protein-Recipes-ebook/dp/B00KDQZH2C

The Tapping Solution for Weight Loss and Body Confidence is a powerful system that releases the emotions and beliefs that hold us back from loving our bodies. I use tapping on a regular basis and have personally benefitted from this powerful method. It's one of the most important practices in my healing arsenal.

Get The **The Ultimate Tapping Solution Guide: Using EFT to tap your way to WEIGHT LOSS, Wealth and Build Body Confidence for Women**

Click Here>> Amazon U.S Link>> http://www.amazon.com/Ultimate-Tapping-Solution-Guide-Confidence-ebook/dp/B00K6JB97S

Books on Health & Fitness Diets

RECOMMENDED BOOK FOR WEIGHT LOSS AND DIET:

**My 10-Day Smoothie Cleanse & Detox Diet Cookbook: Burn the Fat, Lose weight Fast and Boost your Metabolism for Busy Mom,** Restart your life with this cookbook and experience an amazing transformation of your body and your health. I am really excited for you!

CLICK HERE TO BUY: **http://www.amazon.com/10-Day-Detox-Diet-Cookbook-Metabolism-ebook/dp/B00IRE3CV0**

Get this bestselling Grain Brain Book- **My brain against all grain Cookbook: 61 Easy-to-make Healthy Foods that would help you stick to the Grain-Brain-free Diet!**

Discover The Surprising Truth about Wheat, Carbs, and Sugar--Your Brain's Silent Killers

Amazon US Link: http://www.amazon.com/dp/B00J9DX3X0

Amazon UK Link: http://www.amazon.co.uk/dp/B00J9DX3X0

**The Coconut Diet Cookbook: Using Coconut Oil to Lose weight FAST, Supercharge Your Metabolism & Look Beautiful!**

Link http://www.amazon.com/dp/BooK1IIOGS

Made in the USA
Lexington, KY
04 January 2015